RITUALS
for the BATH

FROM THE
RENAISSANCE WOMEN

KATHY COREY *and* LYNNE BLACKMAN

PHOTOGRAPHS *by* NANCY PALUBNIAK

WARNER ⓦ TREASURES™

PUBLISHED BY WARNER BOOKS
A TIME WARNER COMPANY

Rituals for the Bath contains formulas that use essential oils, dried herbs, and other ingredients that are entirely safe when used externally. However, some individuals may have a sensitivity or allergic reaction to certain contents. Please use caution in the preparation and use of these products.

Copyright © 1995 by Kathy Corey and Lynne Blackman
All rights reserved.

Book design by Julia Kushnirsky

Warner Treasures is a trademark of Warner Books, Inc.

Warner Books, Inc., 1271 Avenue of the Americas, New York, NY 10020

A Time Warner Company

Manufactured in Singapore

First Printing: September 1995

10 9 8 7 6 5 4 3 2 1

ISBN: 0-446-91092-9

There are souls on this earth
who don't stay too long.
They come to teach us what we don't know,
laughter, anger, joy, pain, balance, love . . .
Our Self.
We dedicate this work to Jena Corey,
the spirit of this book.

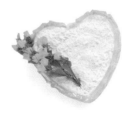

We do not write alone. This book has
been woven from the love and support of our
husbands, family, and friends.

Nurturing and giving come from the heart. They embody the essence of who we are. Developing our ability to give and receive puts us intimately in touch with ourselves. Practicing the art of giving encourages us to rethink our values and develop a fresh way of seeing old things. Sharing gifts with others, with ourselves and with the earth is a way of caring for our souls.

Rituals are essential to a life well lived. They validate the routine of our lives and add mystery and excitement to the ordinary happenings of our days. We recognize ourselves and our families and our relationship to the world through them. They are as ancient as mankind.

Bathing is one of nature's oldest and purist rituals. Water links us to the primordial. The bath is an historical and religious tradition that has survived and evolved in cultures around the world. We bathe to relax, cleanse and beautify our bodies. We bathe to pamper ourselves and feel good.

Rituals for the Bath celebrates the practical and spiritual beauty of bathing with delightful gifts and simple ceremonies. Our easy, inexpensive recipes use natural ingredients for making a full range of bath products with pretty packaging ideas. We adapt the latest aromatherapy formulas and offer fresh and timely rituals for you to share.

The Renaissance Women
Kathy and Lynne

Ritual and tradition make the ordinary in life eternal. They are a profound expression of our humanity and our connection to the mysterious.
– The Renaissance Women

CONTENTS

AUTHOR'S NOTE

Nothing is more exasperating than recipes that don't work. While researching *Rituals for the Bath* we tested hundreds of recipes from dozens of sources. The formulas we have chosen are the best. They work well and are easy to make. Our sincere thanks to the international community of aromatherapists and natural cosmetic experts who contributed their practical knowledge to the making of this book.

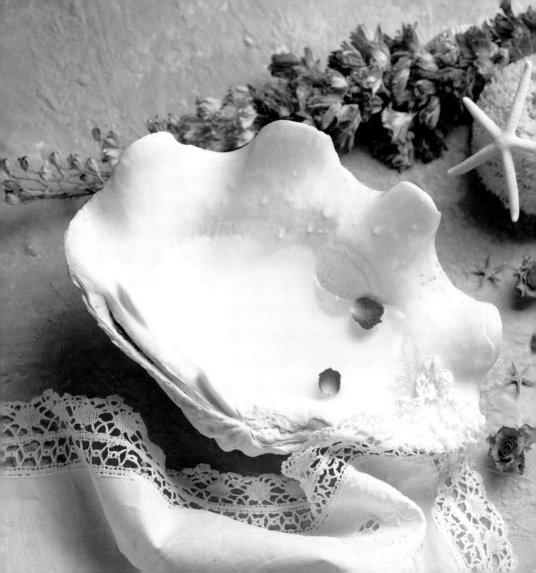

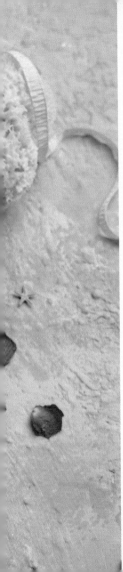

BATHING

Bathing rituals take fascinating forms from the elaborate to the simple. Our inner and outer relationship with water is recognized by all peoples. Water symbolizes our unconscious in modern Jungian dream theory. Primitive societies revere water as mystical and divine. Water holes are sacred to Australian aborigines, who were created in the rainbow mists of the Dreamtime, the time before time began. The Kama Sutra, the erotic fourth-century Sanskrit treatise, instructs lovers in the sensual arts of bathing and exotic massage. Early Roman baths contained theaters and libraries and the hedonistic convenience of forced-hot-air heating. The Caracalla baths of Rome had 1,600 carved marble seats where philosophers and writers could lounge amid the steam and clatter to discuss ideas or read their latest work.

Water is essential to all life. It is a magical elixir that comprises two-thirds of our bodies and two-thirds of our planet. Holding it sacred, playing in it, pleasuring in it are all natural instincts. Mankind, from primitive societies to the most sophisticated, feels an urge to go to water and perform rituals.

Immersing ourselves in water is an affirmation,
a renewal, and a remembrance.
–The Renaissance Women

WATER

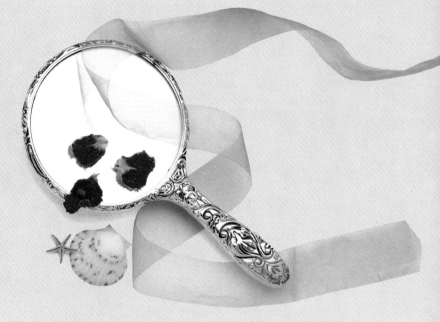

What are you? What am I? Intersecting cycles of water.
earth. air. and fire. that's what I am. that's what you are.
—John Seed and Joanna Macy

Water is the essence and symbol of life. Shimmering in each drop of water, inseparable from the next, dwell our unremembered memories. We experience water's instinctual pull with all of our senses. It speaks to us with a mystical tongue. It whispers to us with gurgles and trickles, or deafens and thunders its message to change our moods. Tides washing timelessly on the continent's shores are the earth's great cosmic clock.

To drink water is to taste translucency. Alone, its flavor is impossible to describe; it is the nectar of life.

Immersing our bodies in water is an affirmation, a renewal, and a remembrance. Its liquid texture caresses ourselves and our senses. Its gentle buoyancy relieves us of the burden of gravity, freeing us to float in that perfect protected space we knew before we were born to air.

AN ELEMENTAL RITUAL

Rituals help us commune with our *selves*. They nourish the quiet, fragile beings we really are. We are so buried in everyday busy-ness that we may not recognize our private selves. Our actions and routines become skewed and meaningless. We act rather than feel; we *do* rather than *be*. Life issues are very difficult to face. We try everything we can to ignore them. Rituals help us reach deep inside and get in touch with our essential natures.

To initiate an elemental ritual, begin by creating a place of safety. Put aside time and give yourself permission to disappear from the world. Combine equal quantities of vivid green kelp and sun-dried sea salt. Pour them into the bottom of the tub, run steaming *hot* water over them, and swirl them into life. Let this fragrant seawater steep. As you strip off your clothes, intentionally remove all pressures. Relax in your elemental bath. Breathe deeply and clear your mind as you would wipe fog from a mirror. Complete your ritual with a cool, freshwater rinse.

When we uncloud the mirrors of our souls we can see farther.
– The Renaissance Women

LIVING WATER RITUALS

Nature provides many opportunities to experience living water.

Walk in the rain. Feel the sheen of newly born moisture on your skin.
Swim in shimmering water by moonlight.
Wade in a rushing stream. Pan for gold.
Stroll in the fog to clear your mind. Drape yourself in its misty fur.
Raft wild rivers. Laugh and let go.
Float naked in the salty summer ocean, rocked by warm tides.
Explore the hidden world of a pond. Make its secrets your own.
Leap from high rocks into a cold lake. Exhilarate your senses.
Rebalance your body in natural mineral springs.
Dabble in muddy puddles with a child.
Sail away!

THALASSOTHERAPY CRYSTALS

Water therapy for tense, tired muscles. Epsom salts have been used for generations to soothe and relax. Double or triple this formula and store the gleaming crystals beside the tub. These salts keep indefinitely.

2	**cups Epsom salts**
6	**drops blue food coloring**
5	**drops each lavender, lemongrass, tea tree, and orange essential oil**

Place salts in a glass bowl. Add food coloring and oils. Mix until salts, color, and oils are blended. Looks striking in a clear glass jar. Dissolve ½ cup (or more) in hot running water.

CYPRESS SALTS

In increasingly popular Indian philosophy there are seven energy centers called chakras. They extend in a vertical line from the head to the base of the spine and affect all the functions of the body. Pine needle and rosemary oil vibrate at the sixth chakra. Pine needle acts upon the adrenal cortex, enhancing our sense of well-being and sharpening the mind. Rosemary awakens the power of the third eye and heightens intuition and remembrance. Cypress stimulates the seventh chakra at the top of the head, opening our meditative energies.

2	cups Epsom salts
6	drops green food coloring
12	drops each cypress, pine, and rosemary essential oil

Place salts in a glass bowl. Add food coloring and oils. Mix until salts, color, and oils are blended. Store in airtight containers. Dissolve 1 cup in hot running water.

RESTORATIVE ROCK SALTS

Sparkling multifaceted crystals that hold their shape as they release fragrance and color into the water.

2	cups coarse rock salt
6	drops yellow food coloring
6	drops each sandalwood, vetiver, and tangerine essential oil
¼	teaspoon glycerin

Place salts in a glass bowl. Add food coloring and oils. Mix until salts, color, and oils are blended. Add glycerin and stir to blend. To use toss ½ cup into hot running water. Give these as gifts in recycled glass containers. Liqueur decanters, spice bottles, and apothecary jars show them off well.

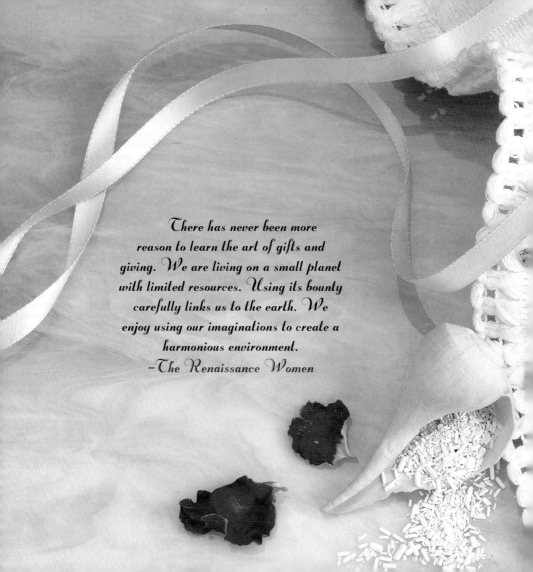

There has never been more reason to learn the art of gifts and giving. We are living on a small planet with limited resources. Using its bounty carefully links us to the earth. We enjoy using our imaginations to create a harmonious environment.

—The Renaissance Women

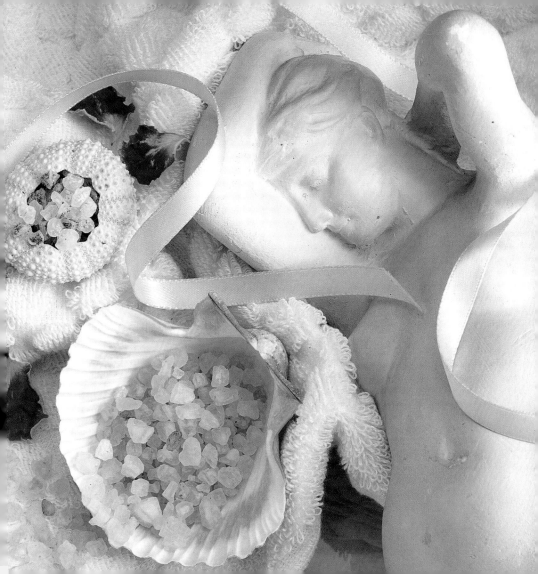

OCEAN EVENING SEA SOAK

This velvety perfumed soak recalls the ocean's evening song and is the color of Homer's wine dark sea.

2	**cups coarse sea or kosher salt**
6	**drops violet food coloring (or 3 drops each red and blue)**
18	**drops violet or heliotrope perfume oil**
¼	**teaspoon glycerin**

Place salts in a glass bowl. Add food coloring and oils. Mix until salts, color, and oils are blended. Add glycerin and stir to blend. Use ½ cup in hot running water. Stop at neighborhood garage sales for antique bottles and unusual containers.

FAMOUS FIZZING SPA BATH

This recipe is a secret from a famous California beauty spa. Soak in tingling world-class luxury!

½	**cup baking soda**
¼	**cup citric or ascorbic acid**
¼	**cup cornstarch**
15	**drops grapefruit essential oil**
5	**drops yellow food coloring**

Mix food colorings together in small glass container. Combine dry ingredients in food processor. Add food coloring and mix well. Add oil and blend. Sprinkle two tablespoons of salts over hot bathwater just before entering tub.

BATH TEMPERATURE

Water temperatures have varied effects on the bather.

Hot baths, in water 100 to 104 degrees Farenheit, eliminate body toxins and muscle soreness.

Warm baths, 90 to 98 degrees Farenheit, are the most soothing and are best for cleansing.

Cold baths, under 75 degrees Farenheit, constrict blood vessels and are used to reduce swelling.

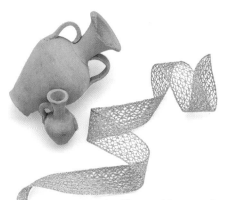

Collecting opens your eyes to the world around you.
Everything you see becomes a potential treasure.
–The Renaissance Women

SHARING

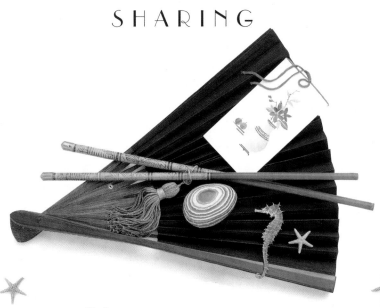

We have learned that inner truths
come to us not only as we sit together in silence,
but as we listen wholeheartedly
to each other speak.
—Sherry Ruth Anderson and Patricia Hopkins

JAPANESE BATHING CEREMONY

Nowhere on earth has the practice of bathing been so thoughtfully and artistically ritualized as in Japan. The Japanese bath is designed to rebalance and center the self, communicate with others, and commune with nature. It is a wholesome, social activity to be shared with family and friends where people come together to exchange daily events in a caring and serene atmosphere. The purpose of the Japanese bath is not to wash the dirt from the body, rather it is to cleanse mind and spirit and experience humanity's age-old relationship with nature.

You can perform a Japanese bath ritual in your own hot tub or Jacuzzi. Choose a clement evening after the sun has set and invite people whose company and conversation you enjoy to share this health-giving *sento*. Ask your friends to bring a kimono or comfortable robe and a large terry-cloth towel.

Set a Japanese mood. Search your cupboards for items with Oriental flair. Hurricane lamps, glassed candles, and colorful lanterns can convert your patio into a Zen garden. Subtle incense burned in flowerpots or bowls of sand will wreathe the night in mystery. Harmonious music is essential: Kitaro, water sounds, or Windham Hill.

Scent your spa with floral salts or a few drops of ginger or balsam oil. Turn off the jets so that your tub becomes a peaceful pond and raise the thermostat. In Japan water is often over 104 degrees. A comfortable zone is 98 to 102 degrees.

Fill woven baskets with loofahs, scrubbers, sponges, and a variety of soaps and gels. You will need to gather several large plastic water buckets, dippers, and a few low stools to sit on.

Prepare a pot of jasmine or green tea as your friends arrive. Plan to serve it outdoors in Japanese teacups to begin your ceremony. Give your guests a place to change into their kimonos and leave their shoes and clothes behind. Fill the plastic buckets with hot water. Take turns sitting on the stools, dip into the buckets, and ladle water over each other. Choose a soap or gel, lather generously, and scrub one another's backs with the loofahs and sponges. Dip again into the buckets and rinse away the lather when you've had enough fun.

Sink slowly into the hot tub, being careful not to submerge too quickly. Go at your own pace until you are neck-deep in the hot water. Feel the heat penetrate down to your bones. Soak and relax for three to ten minutes as stress, tension, and muscle aches dissolve away. Lift yourself out of the tub and air-dry in the cool night for the same amount of time. Alternate the water and air treatments as long as you like. Standing too quickly can make you dizzy. Move slowly.

After the last water session, wrap your dripping body in your dry robe or towel and lie down on the deck or lawn and count the lights in the night sky. Feel how all the hardness has gone from your body, leaving it like voluptuous jelly. Thoughts and impulse come slowly, in cadence with the earth's rhythm.

Refreshments are served after a Japanese bath. When you feel ready, iced beer, juice, mineral water, sake, or wine will taste like nectar, and salty snacks, salads, or sushi will revitalize you.

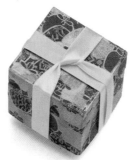

The manner of giving is worth more than the gift.
–Pierre Corneille

APPRECIATION GIFTS

Remember the thrill of your first macaroni-and-glue masterpiece? Your hands immortalized in plaster of Paris? Or construction-paper Christmas ornaments? Making them aroused our inner artist. We gave them to family and friends, bursting with pride, and our creations were displayed with equal enthusiasm. Making gifts and giving of ourselves is what puts quality and richness into our lives.

The best way to brighten someone's day is with a gift of appreciation. We overlook faces we see daily. We live our lives among friendly strangers: the teller at the bank, the checkout person whose line we frequent, the neighbor we wave to on the street, the dog groomer, the dry cleaner, and the librarian. Send these gifts with the letter you have forgotten to answer, to a relative you seldom see, an old school friend, an elderly shut-in, or your child's teacher. Handmade gifts don't have to be perfect. People accept them readily; they are not embarrassed by their cost. It is your thoughtfulness that counts.

Creating and giving handmade gifts is a satisfying personal ritual. Finding materials encourages you to see the world with an artist's eye. Sharing the process with a friend deepens your relationship with laughter and love. Gifts of appreciation bring joy. Stash a variety where you can admire your artistry and give on impulse. Don't wait for an occasion, give them just *because*.

BATH BAGS

Many of our recipes can be packaged in bath bags for an appreciated gift. Sew a bag of colored fabric, order muslin bags through our Source Guide, or tie contents in a handkerchief or washcloth with a pretty ribbon.

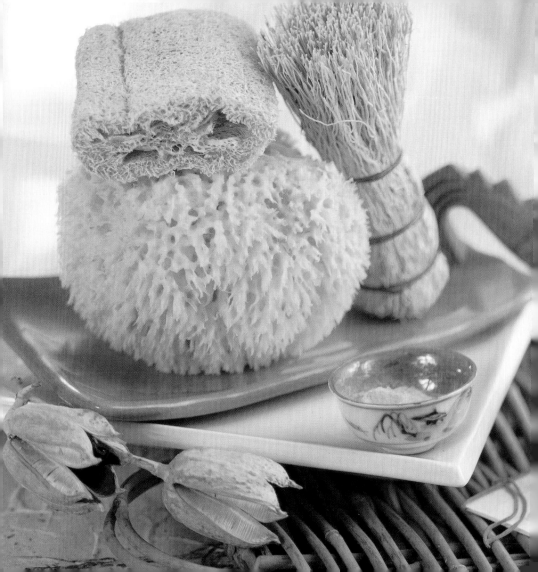

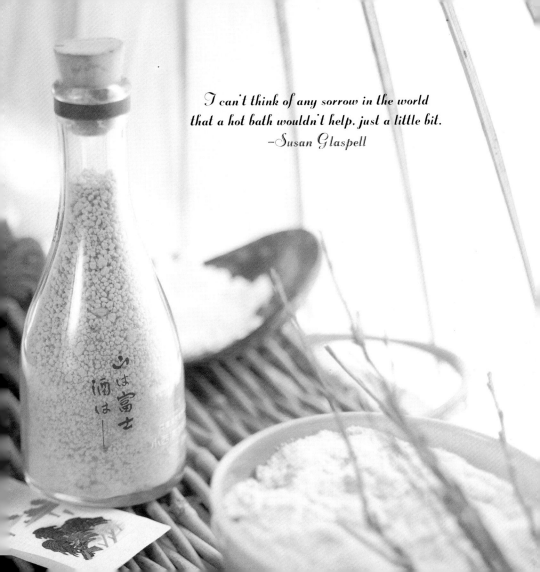

*I can't think of any sorrow in the world
that a hot bath wouldn't help, just a little bit.*
—Susan Glaspell

HONEYSUCKLE SILK BATH

This easy formula will surround you in a cloud of sweetness and alleviate the day's troubles.

2	**cups baking soda**
1	**cup cornstarch**
⅛	**teaspoon honeysuckle perfume oil**
½	**teaspoon yellow food coloring**
½	**teaspoon red food coloring**

Combine dry ingredients in food processor. Add food coloring and mix well. Add oil and blend. Sprinkle ½ cup over hot bathwater just before entering tub.

ORIENTAL FIVE SPICE BATH

This spicy potion is a great gift for the man in your life. Chinese Five Spice can be found at your grocery or Oriental market. It is a licorice-scented combination of anise, cinnamon, ginger, allspice, and cloves.

1	**cup cornstarch**
1	**cup rice flour**
8	**drops musk oil**
8	**drops caramel color**
2	**tablespoons Chinese five spice**

Combine dry ingredients in food processor or blender. Add oil and blend. Add food coloring and mix well. Store in a small sake bottle. Tie on an Oriental spoon. Disperse 2 spoonfuls in hot bathwater just before entering tub.

WHITE GODDESS MILK BATH

Creamy milk baths have softened the bodies of notorious beauties throughout history.

1	**cup cornstarch**
2	**cups dry milk powder**
⅛	**teaspoon almond fragrance oil**

Combine dry ingredients in food processor or blender. Add oil and blend. Add ½ cup to hot bathwater or fill a bath bag with this caressing mixture.

STRAWBERRIES AND CREAM BATH BAG

The gentle buffing action of this luxurious bath bag will leave your skin feeling like satin.

½	**cup oatmeal**
½	**cup powdered milk**
4	**tablespoons almond meal**
15	**drops strawberry perfume oil**

Combine dry ingredients in bowl. Stir to mix well. Add essential oil and blend. Makes three bath bags. Add to tub of running hot water.

Developing our ability to give and receive
puts us intimately in touch with ourselves.
–The Renaissance Women

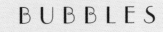

BUBBLES

There is no place like a bath to stretch your soul and listen to your inner voice.

—Seneca

No one knows who invented soap. A colorful, archaic legend attributes its discovery to a pagan ritual. On a rugged cliff above a stony riverbank, chanting worshipers gathered under a storm-blackened moon to make animal sacrifices to their gods over pyres of flaming wood. Raindrops drenched the smoldering fires. Melted animal fats and wood lye, leached from the ashes, mixed together and ran into the river below, creating strands of oily suds. Women coming to wash clothing at the water's edge discovered that the strange yellow substance made their garments whiter and cleaner.

Complexion bars are enriched to soften and moisturize our skin with cocoa butter, olive oil, lanolin, wheat germ, avocado, and glycerin. They are made luxurious with whipped honey and cold cream to smooth, vitamin oils and milk acids to deter aging, and herbs and oatmeal for sensitive-skin care.

Bath collections have expanded to include liquid soaps, gels, and bubble baths that are generally nonirritating and less drying than old-fashioned soap. They do not leave a residue on body or tub and foam and lather splendidly. Liquids and gels are convenient in the shower when time does not permit longer pampering.

A variety of new formulas contain herbal extracts and plant saponins that have been used for hundreds of years in folk practice and traditional medicine. Ecological awareness has made us refocus on nature's gifts. We are in danger of losing so much of our natural world that we have become much more sensitive to the enormous value of our planetary heritage.

Many of us do not want to use animal products on our face and body. Laboratory research is proving many age-old ingredients to be as effective as their animal or chemical equivalents. These alternatives are safer, purer, and kinder to the earth and its inhabitants.

Soaps that were once the province of the wealthy continue to make us feel royal, refreshed, and clean. They were an extravagance only a few could afford. Today brightly wrapped specialty soaps presented in imaginative baskets and boxes are an intelligent gift for a hostess, bride, or friend.

AN EVENING OF RED ROSES

We pass so quickly through the stages of romance that we hardly notice when the flame of love is obscured by the demands of everyday life. The acuteness of the emotions with which we began can be lost in work, errands, and family. Romantic rituals are a way of maintaining and revisiting the intensity that initially drew us together. Rituals keep feelings alive by repeating our romantic patterns. Conscious loving is an art that deserves to be practiced sincerely and often. Daily actions fuel the flame of our relationships.

Anticipation is a delicious part of our red rose ritual. An enticing invitation is the beginning to an evening of intimacy: call him, send him the perfect card, or write a poem on the back of a photo of the two of you laughing together. Set a time and date and mark your calendars.

Your shopping list will include two sumptuous bath towels, a bottle of champagne, Chambord or cassis liqueur, two champagne flutes, your own bubble bath, lots of candles, and six to sixty deep crimson roses.

Set the scene in advance with sensual lighting and passionate music. A few minutes before your lover is due to arrive, place the champagne and glasses on ice next to the tub with the liqueur. To make a Red Rose Royale, pour an inch of liqueur into the flute and add chilled champagne. Top with a rose petal. Fill the tub with steamy water and mountains of frothy bubbles. Undress and wrap yourself in one of the fluffy new towels. Gather your roses. Beginning in your bedroom, pull the petals from the roses and toss them onto the open bed. Scatter a trail of petals from bed to bath. Cover the bubbles with a sprinkling of rose petals. From the tub continue your trail to the door and greet your lover with his towel and your last red rose. Retrace your steps and savor your evening.

The effects of an evening of intimacy will remain in your heart and body through the clutter of a busy week. A single rose on your desk—or your partner's—will transport you to the splendor of your interlude for weeks afterward. Feelings and memories linger long after the rose is gone.

Conscious loving is an art that deserves
to be practiced sincerely and often.
–The Renaissance Women

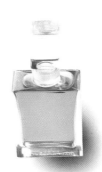

WILD CHERRY BUBBLE BATH

This long-lasting bubble bath produces towering masses of substantial bubbles that are wholesome and mischievous at the same time. Wild Cherry Bubble Bath may also be used as a shower gel or liquid hand soap in your guest bathroom.

¼	**cup glycerin**
1	**cup unscented bubble bath or mild liquid soap**
	(Ivory or Palmolive for sensitive skin)
1	**tablespoon corn syrup**
1 to 1½	**teaspoons cherry perfume oil**
5	**drops red food coloring**

Mix first three ingredients, stirring gently to avoid foaming. Add oils and coloring. Stir to blend. Pour it into decorative stoppered bottles for your friends.

MAGIC RAINBOW BUBBLE BATH

Bath time is an opportunity to switch hats from work to play and change the direction of the day. Bubbles elate. They are water's buoyant laughter. Children love them too. Citrus oils are known for their calming aromatherapy effects. Lavender oil is a harmonizer, and cedarwood is added to improve respiration. This formula is nondrying and suited for sensitive skin.

1	**cup gentle children's liquid soap or shampoo for sensitive skin**
¼	**teaspoon each tangerine, sweet orange, and lime essential oils**
⅛	**teaspoon each lavender and cedarwood essential oils**
5	**drops yellow food coloring (optional)**
3	**drops red food coloring (optional)**

Mix oils and color into shampoo, stirring gently to avoid foaming. Pour in plastic safety bottle for children; a recycled honey-bear squeeze bottle will delight any tot.

VANILLA APRICOT SHOWER GEL

We give this recipe four stars. Vanilla Apricot is warm, rich, and irresistible. A squeeze bottle of amber gel is a his-and-her gift that will keep your friends asking for more.

1	**cup unscented shower gel**
1¾	**teaspoons each vanilla and apricot perfume oils**

Stir oils into shower gel until completely blended. Store away from heat and light. Keeps for up to six months.

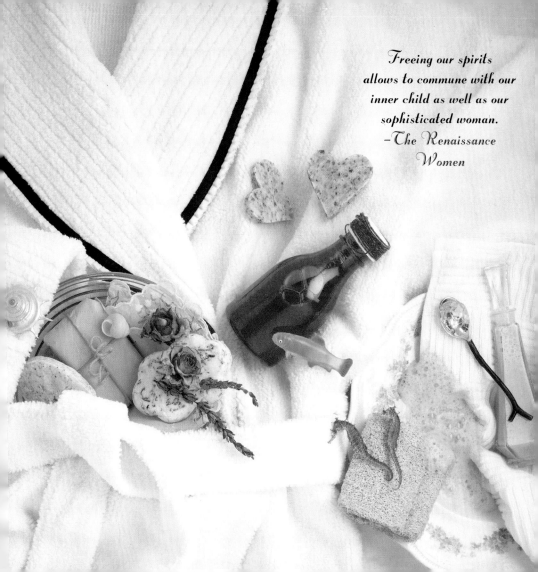

Freeing our spirits allows to commune with our inner child as well as our sophisticated woman.
–The Renaissance Women

DEEP RELIEF SHOWER GEL

Marcel Lavabre pioneered aromatherapy in America. His company, Aroma Vera, sells products that manifest the beauty, elegance, and power of essential oils with respect to the environment. Deep Relief Shower Gel is based on one of their popular formulas.

1   **cup unscented shower gel**
½   **teaspoon each birch and juniper essential oils**
¼   **teaspoon each rosemary, thyme, and vetiver essential oils**

Stir oils into shower gel until completely blended. Use ½ ounce of gel in hot bath to soak and relax. For the shower, apply a small amount to sore muscles.

COTTAGE GARDEN SOAP

Cottage Garden Soap uses dried flowers, petals, or herbs from your garden. Rose petals with tea-rose oil are a delicate alternative. Lemon verbena flowers and oil mixed with lime brings the fresh ambience of the outdoors into your bath.

2   **3 ounce bars grated unscented glycerin soap**
2   **tablespoons cocoa butter or liquid lanolin**
1   **tablespoon dried chamomile flowers**
¼   **teaspoon each chamomile and melissa essential oils**

Melt soap and cocoa butter over low heat, stirring constantly. Remove and add flowers and oils. Stir to blend. Pour into oiled soap molds. Miniature muffin tins or any decorative plastic container can be used. Makes 4 small guest bars. *★For an interesting effect, press a whole dried flower or leaf into the bottom of the mold and pour melted soap over it.*

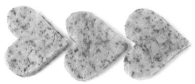

OATMEAL ALMOND SOAP LOG

The white base for this soap also makes a creamy background for brightly colored dried flowers. Try lavender with bachelor's buttons or blue larkspur. Add a spring floral like sweet pea, violet, or honeysuckle. This mixture can be rolled into soap balls and wrapped in foil.

3	**bars shaved lightly scented white complexion soap (e.g., Ivory, Oil of Olay, or Dove)**
3	**tablespoons liquid lanolin**
1½	**teaspoons almond fragrance oil**
1	**tablespoon each almond meal and oatmeal**

Melt soap and lanolin together over low heat, stirring until smooth. Remove from heat and add oil, almond meal, and oatmeal. Stir to blend. Spoon into oiled cardboard juice container. Allow to dry for 2 days. Peel can away. Slice into 1-inch rounds. Trim edges.

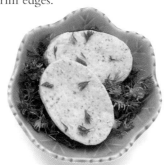

*Give for the sake of giving
and keep it circulating as it flows back.*
–Wayne W. Dyer

AURAS

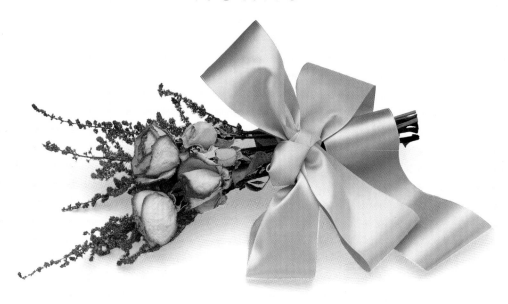

Of all the senses, none surely is so mysterious as that of smell...
Its effects upon the psyche are both wide and deep, at once
obvious and subtle.
—Daniel MacKenzie

A world without scent is unimaginable. Flowers would have no perfume, food would be tasteless. There is a system of scents to warn us of danger, draw us to love, help us tell weather, season, and time of day. We wake to the fragrance of morning coffee, revel in the newness of damp mown grass, wrinkle our noses at the odor of a skunk, choke on exhaust fumes, and sneeze at freshly ground pepper.

Aromatherapy is the ancient practice of using the essential oils of plants to achieve emotional and physical well-being. Essential oils are plant hormones, living cells that circulate in the sap and produce a stimulatory effect on cellular activity. They exist in all parts of the plant in minute quantities. Each essence has a distinctive, potent effect on individuals. In their natural form they are too concentrated to use but when they are diluted have a pleasant odor and beneficial effect. This essential fragrance is the *soul* of the plant.

Plant fragrances generate auras in which our five senses wake in a joint perception or synesthesia where color may be tasted, smell may be seen, and sound may be felt. Our separate senses are inextricably united into a whole, beautifying, healing aura.

Plant essences have been studied for hundreds of years. Their application and the ways in which they affect our psyche and soma are well known. Our Aromatherapy Reference Chart describes popular essential oils and their effects. They can be mixed or used alone. Our Perfume Blending Chart lists additional oils and suggests combinations for making personalized bath and body gifts.

Inexpensive, top-quality unscented lotions, shampoos, soaps, oils, and gels are available in the stores and catalogs listed in our Source Guide. Making a complete line of bath products takes very little time.

Aroma is individual. You can develop a beautiful aura of scent for every personality. Begin your aromatherapy kit with ten or twelve of your favorite oils. No gift is nicer to receive than a perfume that is hand-blended and named especially for you.

AROMATICS

A few drops of essential oil in the tub is still the most ingenuous way to customize your bath.

- Treat your pillows, bed, and bath with atomized spray.
- Put a few drops of fragrance oil in a light ring or directly on an ordinary 100-watt lightbulb. Heat will spread its bouquet through the room.
- Diffusers, which work on small aquarium pumps, are available in aromatherapy and bath catalogs.
- Set a mood with three drops of perfume oil in the hot wax of a burning candle. Oils are inflammable so avoid getting them on the wick.
- Potpourris made of sea glass, unglazed ceramic, or dried botanicals absorb scent and release it gradually.

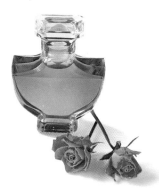

Nothing so swiftly creates an atmosphere of happiness as fragrance. The mind insensibly forgets its cares. and the soul dreams.
– Richard Le Gallienne

AROMATHERAPY REFERENCE CHART

Essential and perfume oils vary in strength and richness from different companies. Quality and price are directly related. Generally the more expensive oils are purer and truer. Adjust quantity to individual taste in all recipes.

Essential oils are extremely concentrated. Do not use directly on skin. Dilute before using. Keep oils away from eyes.

ESSENTIAL OIL	PHYSICAL HEALING POWERS	EFFECTS ON PSYCHE AND EMOTIONS	AROMA AND BLENDING NOTE* *(SEE "PERFUMERY NOTES")
BASIL	alleviates muscle spasms, diuretic	eases anxiety, invigorates, uplifting for mind and intellect	hot, rich, and "green" *top note*
BAY	analgesic, antiseptic increases respiration	invigorates, refreshes	fresh, herbal, hot, and sharp *middle to top note*
BIRCH	alleviates muscle spasms, antiseptic	invigorates, refreshes	woodsy and wintergreen *top note*
CARDAMOM	increases respiration, relieves headaches	aphrodisiac, invigorates, warms and cheers	spicy, warm, and woody *top note*

CHAMOMILE	anti-inflammatory, lubricates dry skin, relieves muscle tightness	aids insomnia, anti-depressant, calms nerves, relaxes	outdoorsy and applelike *top to middle note*
CLARY SAGE	minimizes wrinkles, soothes irritated skin	aids insomnia, antidepressant, calms nerves, eases anxiety	distinctive and pungently herbal *top to middle note*
CORIANDER	combats arthritis and rheumatism, relieves headaches, stimulates circulation	promotes well-being, warms and cheers	spicy, warm and woody *top note*
CYPRESS	breaks down cellulite, diuretic, stimulates circulation	heals the pain of emotional transition, uplifting for mind and intellect	warm and evergreen *middle to base note*
EUCALYPTUS	antiseptic, increases respiration	balances mind, body and spirit; invigorates	sharp and medicinal *top note*
FIR (Needle)	antiseptic, increases respiration	balances mind, body and spirit; uplifting	pure evergreen *middle to base note*
GINGER	combats arthritis and rheumatism, stops motion sickness	clears confusion, comforts loneliness, energizing	strong and spicy *base to middle note*

GRAPEFRUIT	astringent, detoxifier	antidepressant, eases anxiety, use for PMS	fresh citrus *top note*
JUNIPER	antiseptic, breaks down cellulite, detoxifier and diuretic	aids insomnia, calms nerves, sharpens memory	warm and cedarlike *middle to top note*
LAVENDER	antiseptic, enhances skin, rejuvenates, relieves headaches	balances mind, body and spirit; calms nerves, refreshes	clean, refreshing, and sharp *top to middle note*
LEMON	antiseptic, diuretic	inspires optimism, refreshes, warms and cheers	clean and citrusy *top note*
LEMONGRASS	antiseptic, reduces aches and pains, relieves headaches	aids insomnia, calms nerves, sedating	lemony with an herbal edge *top to middle note*
MARJORAM	analgesic, relieves headaches, stimu-lates circulation	aids insomnia, calms nerves	distinctive and pungently herbal *middle note*
MELISSA (Lemon Balm)	relieves headaches, soothes irritated skin	calms nerves, inspires optimism, uplifting	earthy, herbal lemon *middle note*
NUTMEG	analgesic, combats arthritis and rheumatism	invigorates, uplifting for mind and intellect	provocative, sensual spice *base to middle note*

ORANGE (Sweet and Bitter)	disinfectant, enhances skin	bolsters courage, calms nerves, promotes well-being	sweet and citrusy *top note*
PALMAROSA	antiseptic, rejuvenates, soothes irritated skin	calms nerves, refreshes	earthy, herbal lemon *top to middle note*
PATCHOULI	anti-inflammatory, antiseptic, rejuvenates	aphrodisiac, sensual, sharpens memory	musky and earthy *base note*
PEPPERMINT	antiseptic, decongestant, reduces aches and pains	energizing, euphoriant, warms and cheers	cool and minty *middle to base note*
PETITGRAIN	astringent, enhances skin	balances mind, body and spirit; sharpens memory	pleasantly floral, a good neroli substitute *top note*
PINE (Needle)	antiseptic, reduces aches and pains, stimulates circulation	eases anxiety, invigorates, warms and cheers	pure evergreen *middle to base note*
ROSE GERANIUM	improves aging skin, rejuvenates	antidepressant, calms nerves, sharpens memory, uplifting	good rose substitute *middle note*
ROSEMARY	combats rheumatism and arthritis, facilitates hair growth	comforts loneliness, sharpens the memory, uplifting	invigorating and piny *middle note*

SAGE	astringent, facilitates hair growth, rejuvenates	inspires optimism, refreshes, sharpens the memory	sharp and strongly herbal *top note*
SANDAL-WOOD	antiseptic, astringent, improves aging skin, moisturizer	aphrodisiac, balances mind, body and spirit; euphoriant	warm, woody, and exotic *base note*
TANGERINE	breaks down cellulite, detoxifier, diuretic	calms nerves, heals pain of emotional transition	sweeter and warmer than other citrus *top note*
TEA TREE	antifungal, antiseptic, soothes irritated skin	promotes well-being	strong, powerful, and medicinal *top note*
THYME	antiseptic, detoxifier, stimulates circulation	aids insomnia, antidepressant, uplifting	fresh, clean, and herbal *top to middle note*
YLANG-YLANG	improves aging skin, rejuvenates	aphrodisiac, antidepressant, euphoriant	voluptuous, exotic, and floral *middle to base note*

*Exercising our creativity opens us
to a deepening of emotion and feeling of self-worth.*
–*The Renaissance Women*

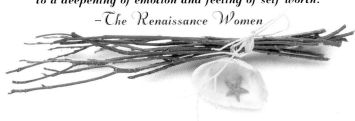

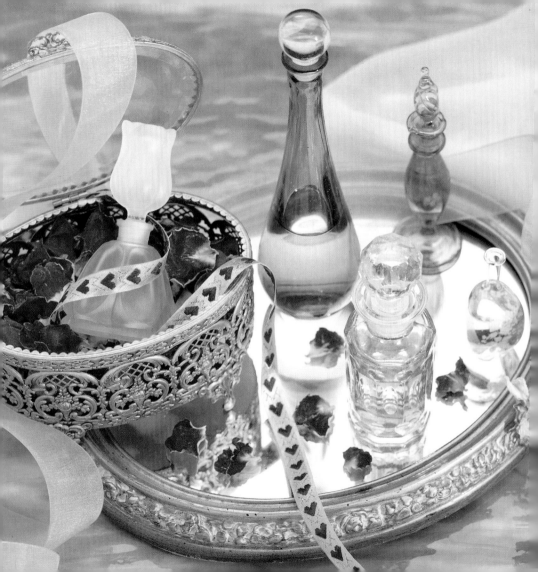

ESSENTIAL OIL BLENDS

Perfume oils can be substituted for the essential oils in these blends, but we prefer them in their pure state.

NEROLI

Christine Malcolm of Santa Fe Fragrance Consultants has blended this emotionally uplifting perfume with rare and precious ingredients.

1	**drop jasmine**
5	**drops neroli**
6	**drops sandalwood**
3	**drops petitgrain**
2	**drops frankincense**
3	**drops ylang-ylang**
1¼	**teaspoons jojoba oil**

Drop all ingredients except jojoba oil into ¼-ounce perfume vial. Add jojoba to fill to top. Cap and shake. Makes an excellent roll-on perfume.

VENUS

Venus is the original perfume, *according to Victoria Edwards of Leydet Aromatics. In ancient India the formula included crushed pearls and honey. It is eloquent and exquisitely balanced.*

¾	**teaspoon sandalwood essential oil**
12	**drops each pure rose and jasmine**
½	**teaspoon jojoba oil**

Place sandalwood, rose, and jasmine in ¼-ounce perfume vial. Add jojoba oil. Cap and shake to blend.

Odour is the story of language, of man's efforts to find words to express emotion and sensation. It is alive with all the senses, indissolubly with taste, with colour, sound and memory, and deeply affected by the psychological phenomenon, the power of suggestion.
–Edward Sagarin

DISPERSING BATH OIL

Turkey red is sulfated castor oil and is the only oil that completely disperses in water. It softens water without leaving a residue on body or tub, making it perfect to use in your spa. Grades of Turkey red oil vary. We like the ones from Aroma Vera or Essentials & Such.

SUMMER SOLSTICE BATHING OIL

Aromatherapist Ixchel Leigh offers this blend for summer rituals. The summer solstice, June 21 is the longest day of the year. During this time of fullness we give thanks for the abundance of all things. We like to extend its use to celebrate each full moon.

6	**drops each ginger and cinnamon essential oils**
10	**drops each clove, nutmeg, and ylang–ylang essential oils**
18	**drops clary sage essential oil**
15	**drops geranium essential oil**
¼	**teaspoon palmarosa essential oil**
½	**teaspoon orange essential oil**
4	**ounces Turkey red oil**

Pour Turkey red oil into bottle. Add essential oils in order given. Blend all oils. Pour ½ cup under running water or add to spa or whirlpool. For a massage oil use half the amount of the listed essential oils to 4 ounces sweet almond oil.

SPORTIF BATHING OIL

This formula is inspired by an outstanding mixture from L'Herbier de Provence. Founded twenty years ago in the south of France, this natural-products company now has stores across the United States.

4	**ounces Turkey red oil**
1	**ounce pine-needle essential oil**
½	**ounce each peppermint and rosemary essential oils**

Blend all oils. Bottle and store in a cool place for two weeks to integrate essences. Pour ½ cup under running water or add to spa or whirlpool. It disperses completely and will not clog jets.

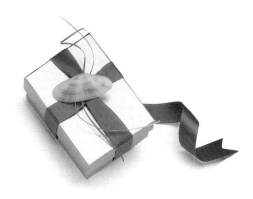

PERFUMERY NOTES

Blending your personal scent is sweet and simple. You can summon any scene or mood: a meadow of delicate alpine flowers, summer rain, breezes sweeping across a Tahitian lagoon, ripe strawberries or midnight adventures in the Casbah.

Perfumers express scents in the language of music. Harmony is achieved through the integration of notes. Base notes are the stabilizers, the heavy bottom of the formula, and are often gums, roots, and resins. They last for more than a week. Middle or heart notes are usually floral and linger for two or three days. They build an aromatic bridge to the sharp or citrusy top notes. These light notes are the ones you smell first, and they evaporate in one day.

Each note may be composed of several oils. Mix your middle notes first. Choose a complimentary base and blend your middle notes into it. Finish by selecting your top notes. Combine these and add them to your perfume oils. A well-balanced composition consists of one part base to two parts middle to four parts top note.

Essential oils (EO) are natural plant extracts. Some plant oils do not yield the aroma we normally associate with them or their extraction is extremely complicated and expensive. Perfume oils (PO) are synthetic substitutes.

FOR PERFUME: Add ½ ounce of base to ¼ ounce of oil.

FOR EAU DE TOILETTE OR SPRAY: Add two ounces of diluent to ½ ounce perfume oil.

FOR COLOGNE: Add four ounces of diluent to ½ ounce of oil.

EQUIVALENCY CHART

DROPS	TEASPOONS	OUNCES
25	¼	
50	½	
	¾	⅛
	1½	¼
	3	½
	6	1

PERFUME BLENDING CHART

Essential and perfume oils vary in strength and richness from different companies. Quality and price are directly related. Generally the more expensive oils are purer and truer. Adjust quantity to individual taste in all recipes.

See Aromatherapy Reference Chart for additional fragrances.

OIL	EO OR PO	NOTE	AROMA	BLENDS WITH
ALMOND	PO	middle	fruity, intense, sweet	stands alone; clove, ginger, nutmeg
BALSAM	EO	base	rich, warm, vanillalike	bergamot, jasmine, lemon, mandarin, and rosewood
BERGAMOT	EO	top	citrus, cool, fresh	most florals, cypress, juniper and patchouli
CARNATION	PO	middle	floral, oriental, spicy	most citrus and spices, heliotrope, patchouli, musk

CEDARWOOD	EO	base	fresh, resinous, spicy	jasmine, hyacinth, neroli, rose, sandalwood, vetiver
CHERRY	PO	middle	fresh, fruity, sweet	stands alone; most citrus, almond, vanilla
CINNAMON	EO	base to middle	Oriental, spicy, warm	most spices, frankincense, myrrh, rose, violet
COCONUT	PO	middle	rich, sweet, tropical	gardenia, vanilla, ylang-ylang
CLOVE	EO	middle	powerful, sharp, spicy	most spices, citrus, peppermint, rosemary
FRANGIPANI	PO	middle	sensual, sweet, tropical	heliotrope, neroli, rose, sandalwood
FRANKIN-CENSE	EO	base	oriental, resinous, sharp	basil, citrus, lavender, pine, rose geranium
GARDENIA	PO	middle	powerful, rich, sensual	stands alone; heliotrope, musk, strawberry
HELIOTROPE	PO	base to middle	fruity, sugary, sweet	carnation, neroli, violet
HONEY-SUCKLE	PO	middle	delicate, feminine, sweet	stands alone; musk, neroli, orange, sandalwood
JASMINE	EO/PO	middle	heavy, musky, sensual	lily of the valley, musk, rose, sandalwood, strawberry

LEMON VERBENA	EO/PO	top	fresh, lemony citrus, sharp	most florals
LILAC	PO	middle	feminine, intense, sweet	stands alone; heliotrope, musk, rose, violet
LILY OF THE VALLEY	PO	top to middle	delicate, feminine, floral	stands alone, lavender, musk, sandalwood, violet
LIME	EO	top	citrus, cool, sharp	most florals, orange, petitgrain, rose geranium
MAGNOLIA	PO	middle	heavy, powerful, sweet	stands alone; honeysuckle, musk, sandalwood
MANDARIN	EO	top	rich, sweet, warm, citrus	most spices, rose, ylang-ylang
MANGO	PO	middle	fresh, fruity, tropical	bergamot, cedar, citrus, musk, neroli, vanilla
MUSK	PO	base	complex, Oriental, vanillalike	jasmine, narcissus, rose, tuberose, violet
MYRRH	EO	base	intense, resinous, sharp	citrus, lavender, pine, sandalwood
NARCISSUS	PO	middle	feminine, floral, light	heliotrope, mandarin, musk, neroli, sandalwood
NEROLI	EO	middle	orange blossom, rich, sweet	most citrus and florals, clary sage, lavender, rose, violet

PEACH	PO	middle	fruity, sugary, sweet	stands alone, gardenia, jasmine, sandalwood, violet
ROSE	EO/PO	middle	best known of all florals, complex, rich	stands alone, florals, clove, cinnamon, jasmine, musk
STRAWBERRY	PO	middle	fruity, light, smells like summer	bergamot, gardenia, jasmine, lime, musk, vanilla, violet
SWEET PEA	PO	top to middle	delicate, feminine, floral, light	lemon verbena, mandarin, musk, vanilla
TUBEROSE	EO/PO	middle	intense, rich, sensual, sweet	carnation, petitgrain, rose geranium, sandalwood
VANILLA	EO/PO	base	complex, rich, sensual, warm	most spices, bergamot, jasmine, neroli, ylang-ylang
VETIVER	EO	base	earthy, musky, spicy, woody	frankincense, sandalwood, violet, ylang-ylang
VIOLET	PO	top to middle	feminine, floral, light	cedar, cinnamon, clove, heliotrope, musk, strawberry

Sweet perfumes work immediately upon the spirits for their refreshing: sweet healthful ayres are special preservatives to health, and therefore much to be prised.
– Ralph Austen

RENAISSANCE PERFUME BLENDS

When we compose a Renaissance perfume for a friend, we sit quietly, close our eyes, and match the fragrances we imagine with his or her personality. We bottle some of this signature perfume and add the rest to unscented bath, body, and hair products. *Voilà!* An instant line of coordinated gifts.

AMAZONIA	CITRINE	ECLIPSE MEN'S COLOGNE	MOON SHADOWS
20 drops each:	4 drops each:	10 drops each:	10 drops each:
vanilla, coconut	marjoram, bay, vetiver, benzoin, patchouli, myrrh	sandalwood, vetiver	jasmine, carnation
½ teaspoon each:	6 drops each:	20 drops each:	20 drops each:
gardenia, ylang-ylang	carnation, rose geranium, ylang-ylang, cinnamon, jasmine	frangipani, grapefruit, bergamot	coriander, petitgrain, neroli
	20 drops:		
	sweet orange		

Place oils in a ½-ounce perfume vial or jar in order given. Shake to blend. Add perfume base to fill bottle. Cap and shake again. Let sit overnight to marry scents.

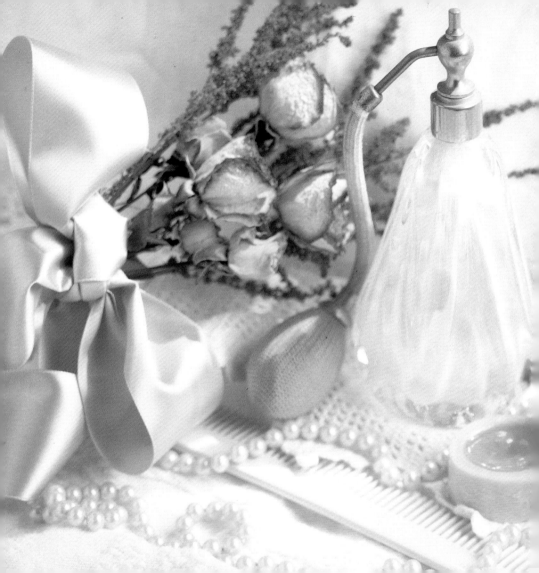

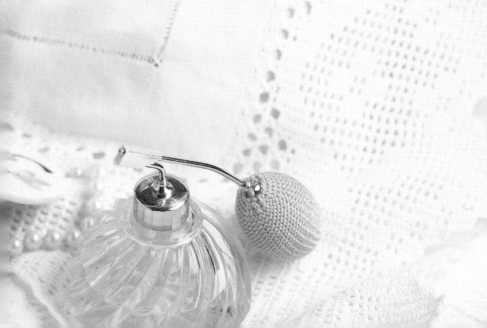

The core of a celebration speaks to the hearts of all humankind—
in all times and in all places.
It speaks the symbolic language of the soul
and is hardly ever practical. but more poetic. playful. prayerful. . . .
—Gertrud Mueller Nelson

BASES

Perfume bases or diluents are added directly to fragrance oils to make a perfume, toilet water, or cologne. See Perfumery Notes for proportions.

OIL BASE: These are heavier, thicker, and richer. We recommend jojoba oil for the smoothest blend, but sweet almond, apricot kernel, or avocado oil can be used.

ALCOHOL BASE: For a lighter, long-lasting blend. Perfumer's diluent can be ordered from our Source Guide. A home mixture can be made by blending 3 teaspoons of odorless 90-proof grain alcohol or vodka with 1 ½ teaspoons liquid vegetable glycerin.

SOLID PERFUME: A great way to travel with perfume. Ships well and makes an unusual gift. It melts onto the skin when applied. Solid perfume requires more essential oil to hold the scent. Adjust recipes to your nose. Heat 3 teaspoons grapeseed oil in the microwave. Melt ½ teaspoon beeswax and add to hot oil. Stir to blend. Allow to cool slightly. Add ½ to ¾ teaspoon fragrance oil and mix well. Pour into container or small jar. Will harden when cool.

Our passion to nurture and create is fundamental.
–The Renaissance Woman

AROMATHERAPY ROOM AND PILLOW MISTS

Don't be tied to commercial room deodorizers. Create an aromatherapy mist that suits your personality and decor. A dusting of spray on your sheets and pillows will forever change the way you dream.

SINGLE SCENT SPRAYS	CHRISTMAS CHEER	STRAWBERRY TREE
1 teaspoon: (Choose one essential oil:) lemongrass rose geranium tangerine sage eucalyptus melissa (Choose one floral:) magnolia heliotrope sweet pea tuberose	**½ teaspoon each:** fir needle, tangerine, orange **20 drops:** cinnamon **10 drops each:** bay, cedarwood, myrrh **5 drops each:** cardamom, clove, nutmeg, ginger	**¼ teaspoon:** juniper **½ teaspoon each:** tangerine, orange **15 drops:** strawberry **10 drops:** cinnamon **5 drops each:** bay, cedarwood **2 drops each:** clove, nutmeg, ginger

Mix oils in 2-ounce spray bottle. Fill to top with diluent. Cap and shake.

BOTANICALS

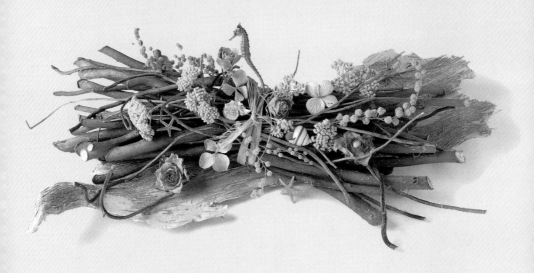

Some things will never change . . .
–Thomas Wolfe

Botanical treatments are ancient and universal. Throughout history the innate properties of flowers and herbs have been discovered, tested in folk use, and gradually classified. This precious knowledge has been shared, and today we appreciate the value of an abundant variety of botanicals.

There are four easy ways to use botanicals in the bath: float them in your tub, put them in bath bags, infuse them in water the way you make a cup of tea, or add their essence directly to your bath.

That which is not celebrated, that which is not ritualized,
goes unnoticed, and in the long run
those feelings and happenings will be devalued.
–Zsuzsanna E. Budapest

CASTING YOUR FATE UPON THE WATERS

We have a science for everything, but some things—like affairs of the human heart—lie beyond logic or sense. They respond better to magic. They answer to feeling, to intuition. A medieval English folktale suggests naming rose petals for your lovers and floating them upon water. The one that remains afloat the longest is sure to be your true love.

There is no better place to solve matters of the heart than in the bath. To cast your fate upon the waters you will need a rose of exceptionally pleasing color. Browse among lavender, peach, pink, or yellow and let one choose you. Fill your tub with warm water and add ten drops of mood-enhancing oil.

Ylang-ylang, gardenia, lilac, frangipani, and jasmine are richly evocative florals. Fragrance may be matched to color. Lemon suits a yellow blossom, peach compliments a peach rose, and apricot flatters coral. Be sensitive to your feelings.

Enter the bath with your flower and pause to appreciate the pleasure and security of the scented water. Remove the petals from the rose's heart and hold them in your cupped hands. Concentrate on the most immediate emotional dilemma in your life. Cast the petals into air and watch them fall on the smooth surface of the water. Choose one with your mind's eye. Ask it a question and remain very still. Keep your attention on the fateful petal. If it floats toward you, the response to your emotional problem is a positive one, a yes. If it moves away, the response is not favorable, a no. If the flower drifts to the side the fates have not yet decided.

Awakening our talents is a way of touching the grace that resides in each of us and of unleashing the energy to create and give through knowing more about ourselves.
–The Renaissance Women

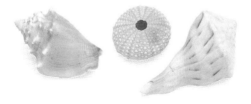

Water is the most healing of all remedies, and the best of all cosmetics.
–Arab Proverb

HERBAL INFUSIONS, BATH BAGS, AND FACIAL STEAMS

Botanical baths with dried herbs and flowers are used to develop depth and wisdom, lull one to sleep, refresh and energize, or soothe and relax. Make an infusion with these therapeutic combinations or place them in a bath bag and add them to a tub of hot water.

Aromatherapist Kathryn McCarthy suggests creating a facial steam tent by draping a bath towel over your head and placing a bowl of steaming herbs below. The trapped herbal vapors will open and cleanse every pore to help you attain a beautiful complexion.

SPIRITUAL	KATHRYN McCARTHY'S SLEEPYTIME	ENERGIZING	RELAXING
lavender rosemary melissa	chamomile marjoram lemon peel 5 drops each: tangerine and rose geranium essential oils	sage thyme basil grapefruit peel	comfrey linden flower catnip lemon verbena 5 drops: lavender essential oil

BATH BAG: Place 1 tablespoon of each ingredient in bath bag. Add essential oil.

INFUSION: 1 tablespoon of each dry ingredient and four cups of water. Place herbs in heat-proof container. In separate pot, bring water to boil. Pour over herbs. Cover and let steep 2 hours or overnight. Strain into bottle. Add essential oils. Keeps up to 3 days in refrigerator. To use, pour entire mixture into hot bathwater.

FACIAL STEAM: Place 1 tablespoon of each ingredient in bowl. Pour steaming water over herbs. Add essential oils. Use as suggested above.

NATURE'S KALEIDOSCOPE GIFT OIL

This colorful, artistic decanter of bath oil contains dried materials, loosely arranged so that floating spaces appear between them. It is a spectacular house-warming gift that can be displayed on the edge of the tub for months. The clear oil catches the light and magnifies the vivid botanicals suspended inside, giving the effect of stained glass.

> **Dried cones, pods, twigs, grasses, vine tendrils, rose hips and petals, statice, lamb's ears, nigella, baby's breath, larkspur, and everlastings**
>
> **7   ounces light oil—sweet almond, castor, canola, apricot, grapeseed or a combination**
>
> **1   tablespoon vitamin E oil**
>
> **1   teaspoon lilac or lily of the valley floral oil**

Arrange dried materials in a tall, thin 8-ounce bottle with a wide mouth. Combine oils in a separate container and pour them slowly into bottle containing dried materials. If necessary, add extra oil to fill to top. Cap or cork tightly. Add 2 tablespoons of oil to a full tub. Oil will float lightly on top of the water and coat and scent your skin as you leave the tub. This is also a lovely massage oil.

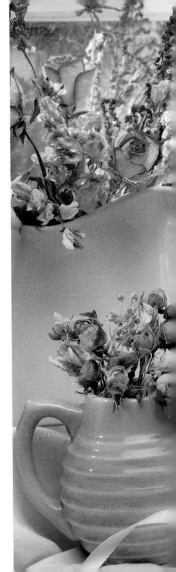

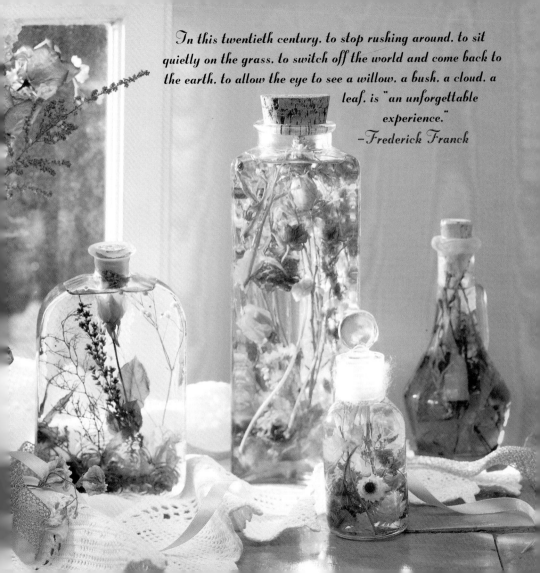

In this twentieth century, to stop rushing around, to sit quietly on the grass, to switch off the world and come back to the earth, to allow the eye to see a willow, a bush, a cloud, a leaf, is "an unforgettable experience."
—Frederick Franck

RARE EARTH

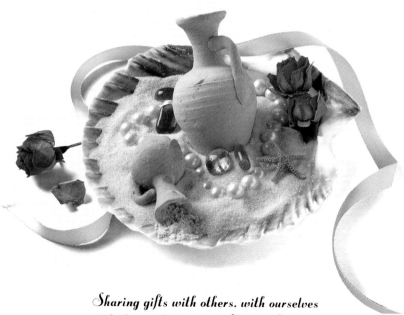

Sharing gifts with others, with ourselves
and with the earth is a way of caring for our souls.
—The Renaissance Women

Nature's first cosmetics are natural, fine-grained crystalline minerals formed millions of years ago when our planet was young. Topaz, tourmaline, feldspar, and glittering flakes of mica and quartz crushed beneath the earth's crust for eons have been transformed by time and nature into precious and therapeutic clays.

Mankind has always ascribed healing power to fine earths. Arenation, the covering of the body in sea sand or warm earth near a hot spring, is a primitive bathing ritual. Clays have been used as medicines and adornments by the learned priests of Egypt, in the opulent court of Kublai Khan, and by the original physicians of classical Greece.

Modern aromatherapists believe clays have positive rejuvenating and anti-aging properties. Clays are an excellent insulation for the skin and are highly absorbent. They are beneficial as astringents and clean without itching. Clays combine synergeristically with essential oils. They improve blood flow and remove dead cells and impurities from the skin.

Cosmetic clays have different mineral contents and come in many colors: subtle green from France, robust red from Morocco, and white from China, Canada, and the United States. *Ganchi*, a yellow clay, is applied to the skin in India to protect from the heat of the sun. Iron-rich red clays are a gift from the volcanoes that altered our continents. Fine ash from their eruptions, drifting on the wind, dusted the entire surface of the globe. White kaolin is a corruption of Kau-ling, or High Ridge Hill, in Kiangsi province of southeastern China where it was first mined. A French Jesuit missionary sent it to Europe in the eighteenth century and introduced porcelain and fine *china* to the Western world.

Exclusive international spas use mineral clays and organic muds to heal and beautify. Rare earths are an irreplaceable ingredient in face powders, makeup, natural deodorant, masks, and most modern cosmetics. They are remarkably inexpensive, readily available, and easy to work with at home.

If women are to pioneer a new way of embodying spirit
in the world today, one thing seems certain:
we must listen to the deep source of wisdom within ourselves
and tell the truth about our lives and what we are learning.
—Sherry Ruth Anderson and Patricia Hopkins

CRYSTALS AND COLOR

Crystals and gems are treasures from the earth. Their vibrational energies heighten our moods and impact our health and well-being. Fact and fancy about crystals and color exist for every expression of daily life. Each day of the week, each month of the year, and each sign of the zodiac has its own crystal and color.

Red is the color of Aries and Scorpio. The healing stones for these signs are jasper, garnet, and aragonite. They radiate love, vigor, and strength.

Yellow shines for Libra and Taurus. Citrine, topaz, and tiger's eye glow under this sign. They signify charm, confidence, joy, and comfort.

Orange warms the house of Leo. Lion signs are attracted to smoky quartz, amber, and carnelian for their encouragement, kindness, and stimulation.

Green soothes the water sign of Cancer with serpentine, malachite, and tourmaline, which defends against negative thoughts. These serene stones bestow energy, growth, and luck.

Blue cools Capricorn, Aquarius, and Pisces. The attributes of blue are intrinsic in sodalite, amazonite, and azurite. They bring serenity, sincerity, and health.

Purple shadows people born in Gemini, Virgo, and Sagittarius. They are drawn to amethyst, lepidolite, and rose quartz which give them power and ease tension and sadness.

The easiest way to choose minerals and gems is by color. Select crystals and stones that appeal to you emotionally. Crystals are stunning in a bathroom where mirrors, glass, and water reflect their many facets. Colored crystals are a focus point for peaceful meditation. They may be scented with any of the fragrance oils in our charts. Match the healing powers and emotional effects of the oils to the crystals. Scented gemstones in an open bowl make a sparkling glass-garden potpourri. Choose a birthday crystal for a friend from this list. Give it as a good-luck talisman with a lettered card of crystal lore.

Rekindling our natural artist allows us to experience
all the colorful aspects of our inner radiance.
– The Renaissance Women

REJUVENATING CLAY FACIAL MASK WITH AHA

Tropical papaya is one of the best natural sources of alpha-hydroxy acids. Our rejuvenating formula combines golden papaya, rich in AHA, fine cosmetic clay, and the ageless healing properties of aloe vera to peel away the accumulating effects of time, leaving skin softer and glowing. Good for all types of skin.

- ¼ **medium-size ripe papaya**
- 1½ **teaspoons aloe vera gel**
- 4 **tablespoons green or white French cosmetic clay**

Place papaya in blender or food processor. Blend until smooth. Add aloe vera gel and blend. Add clay and process until creamy. Makes two masks. Apply to face and neck and leave on for 20 minutes. Rinse with cool water. Will keep in refrigerator for up to five days.

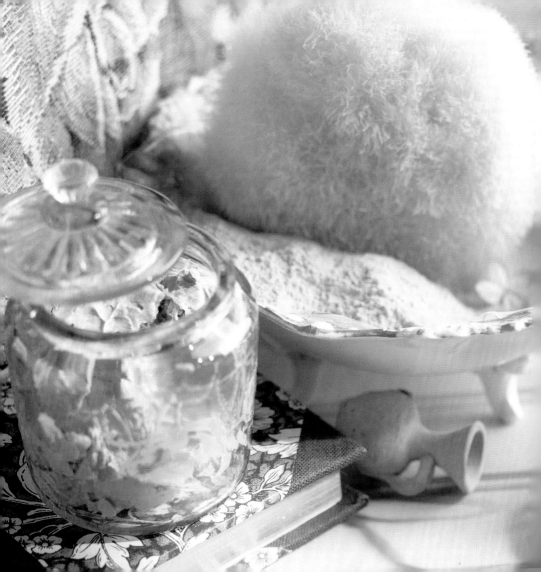

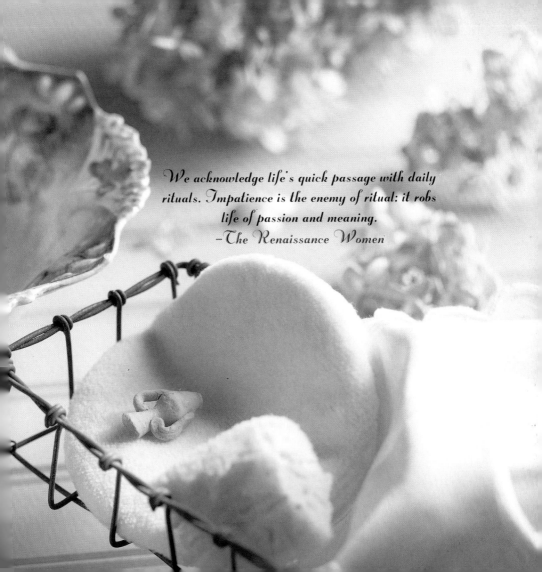

We acknowledge life's quick passage with daily rituals. Impatience is the enemy of ritual: it robs life of passion and meaning.
—The Renaissance Women

ESSENCE BODY AND FACE MASK

Clay masks help remove impurities from the skin. This recipe is based on a formula from Essence AromaTherapy. It is particularly good for dry or mature skin.

2	**tablespoons instant oatmeal**
1	**tablespoon rose or red Moroccan clay**
1	**tablespoon yogurt**
1	**teaspoon jojoba oil**
½	**teaspoon honey**
1	**drop each frankincense, sandalwood, and rose essential oil**

Mix the oatmeal, clay, jojoba, honey, and yogurt together in a small bowl. Add the essential oils and blend well. Thin with a little water if necessary. Apply to face and neck and leave on for 15 minutes. Triple recipe for a body mask and leave on for 25 minutes. Wash off with warm water.

CITRUS BLOSSOM BODY POWDER

The idea for this organic body powder comes to us from Moon River Naturals in Eugene, Oregon. This gentle powder is great on a hot, muggy day or after a bath or shower.

¾	**cup cornstarch**
⅛	**cup arrowroot powder**
1½	**teaspoons bentonite clay (optional)**
2	**teaspoons finely ground calendula flowers**
2	**teaspoons finely ground dried orange peel**
10	**drops ylang-ylang essential oil**
20	**drops grapefruit essential oil**

Combine all ingredients except oils in large bowl. Blend thoroughly. Add essential oils and mix well. Give in a cut-glass candy dish with an oversize powder puff.

LAVENDER DUSTING POWDER

Lavender is the flower of devotion. Ancients believed that a person who wore lavender would be able to see ghosts.

⅓	**cup white kaolin clay**
⅓	**cup arrowroot powder**
⅓	**cup cornstarch**
4	**drops each lavender, clary sage, and mandarin essential oils**

Combine dry ingredients in blender. Add oils and blend. An antique saltshaker is a novel way to dispense body powders.

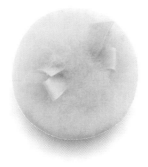

*Ritual and myth are like seed crystals of new patterns
that can eventually reshape culture around them.*
–Starhawk

LOVING MASSAGE

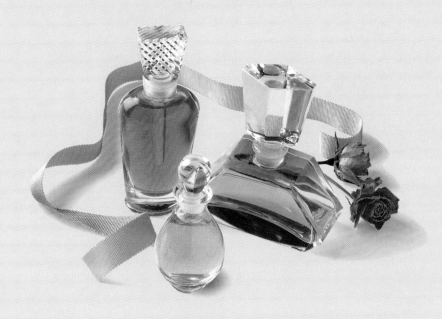

The body is a sacred garment.
—Martha Graham

Massage is an intimate means of communication between partners. It is a way of getting to know and experience our beloved's body through the sensation of touch. Caring touch expands our boundaries. Physical tension is often formed by emotional pain. We hold trauma, anxiety, and fear in constricted body patterns. Emotions are stored like memories in the mute depths of our being. To be able to release them requires mutual understanding, acceptance, and trust. In loving massage, tender hands move with sensitivity and respond to the silent signals of the body, releasing ingrained physical and psychic constrictions.

Loving massage is an interactive relationship from which both giver and receiver benefit equally, both are equally blessed. The more we open to either role, the more we learn about ourselves and our partners. Healing occurs on many levels; romantic massage is a lovely path to intimacy.

Touch is endless lovemaking joining two people in sensory union. Ancient Tantric teachings invoke massage as a sacred art to intensify connectedness. Warmed, scented oils applied to the body increase energy flow. They penetrate with healing effect to open blocked psychic and physical channels. Releasing buried emotional scars allows us to love without barriers.

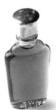

For one human being to love another: that is perhaps the
most difficult of all our tasks. the ultimate. the last test and proof.
the work for which all other work is but preparation.
— Rainer Maria Rilke

Everything in the universe flows.
You can't get ahold of water by clutching it.
Let your hand relax. and you can experience it.
— Wayne W. Dyer

VELVET TOUCH MASSAGE OIL

Innocently erotic. Your partner will appreciate the intricate undertones in this light oil.

- ¼ **teaspoon cardamom essential oil**
- ½ **teaspoon each carnation, jasmine, narcissus, and rose fragrance oils**
- ½ **teaspoon vitamin E oil**
- 8 **ounces sweet almond or grapeseed oil**

Place sweet almond or vegetable oil in plastic squeeze bottle. Add oils and vitamin E. Stir or shake to blend. Let sit overnight. Keeps well when stored away from heat and light, or refrigerate. Warm in microwave with lid removed.

REBALANCING MASSAGE OIL

Our rebalancing formula eases tired muscles after a strenuous workout or training session. Everyday aches and pains will melt away and respiration will improve as it penetrates and warms.

- ¼ **teaspoon each lavender and clary sage essential oils**
- ½ **teaspoon each rose geranium and grapefruit essential oils**
- ½ **teaspoon vitamin E oil**
- 8 **ounces sweet almond oil**

Place sweet almond oil in bottle. Add essential oils and vitamin E oil. Stir or shake to blend.

*Practicing the art of giving encourages us to rethink our
values and to develop a fresh way of seeing old things.*
– The Renaissance Women

TROPICAL DREAM BODY BUTTER

Spread this butter on the body of your choice.

3	**teaspoons beeswax**
¼	**cup sweet almond oil**
¼	**cup glycerin**
1	**teaspoon each mango and peach perfume oil**
3	**drops each red and yellow food coloring**

Melt beeswax in pan. In separate pan, heat almond oil and glycerin. Stir in beeswax. Remove from heat. Place in bowl. Whip with an electric mixer or whisk until well blended. Add oils and food coloring, mixing well. Allow to cool slightly. Whip until cool and thick. Note: placing bowl in large bowl of ice water speeds process. Spoon into jars.

TRADE WINDS BODY LOTION

Comptoir Sud Pacifique's line of fine French fragrances takes its wearers to far-away places and brings paradise into their everyday lives. Our Trade Winds Body Lotion is inspired by their philosophy.

1	**cup unscented lotion**
10	**drops each musk, peach, mango, lemon, lime, grapefruit, bergamot, bitter orange, and tangerine oils**
5	**drops mandarin oil**

Place lotion in container. Make depression in center. Drop oils into depression and stir until completely blended. Pot in small jars and keep on hand for favorite friends.

You are your own miracle, but it takes you to prove it—to experience the wonder of your self.
– Ron Fletcher

PEPPERMINT FOOT MASK

Zia Cosmetics combines the latest innovations in body care with botanical ingredients. Like stepping into clean, wet beach sand, this foot mask exfoliates and refreshes tired feet. The tingling light-footed sensation lasts for hours.

½	**cup oatmeal**
½	**cup cornmeal**
½	**cup coarse salt**
½	**cup mild or unscented lotion**
4	**tablespoons aloe vera gel**
12	**drops peppermint essential oil**

Place oatmeal, cornmeal, and salt in bowl. Stir to blend. Add lotion and aloe vera gel. Mix well. Add peppermint oil and blend. Place in footbath or basin large enough for both feet. Pour warm water into second large basin until half full. Sit in a comfortable chair. Slide feet into foot mask. Beginning at toes, massage between toes and up to top of foot. Massage ankle and heel. Work back under arch and finish at toes. Massage for 5 to 10 minutes. Place foot into basin of warm water and rinse off, one at a time. Massage dry with thick terry towel. **FOR LEGS AND BODY:** Triple recipe. Sit in tub or shower. Begin at toes. Massage feet thoroughly. Massage up body using circular motion. Rinse under warm water.

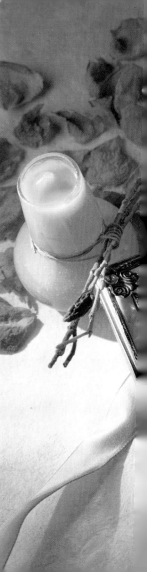

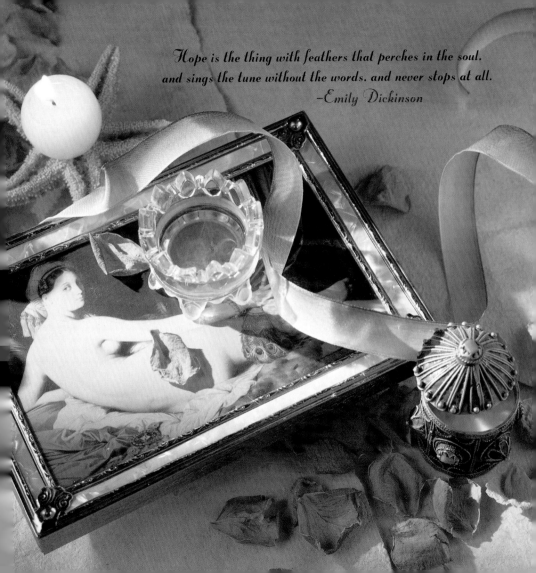

Hope is the thing with feathers that perches in the soul,
and sings the tune without the words, and never stops at all.
—Emily Dickinson

TAKING TIME

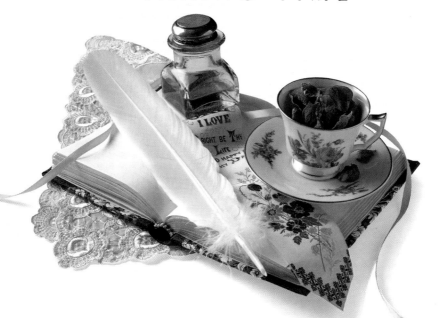

We return to the simple, to childhood, to
innocence, as we draw upon our instincts to view ourselves
anew and establish our commitment to the process of
growth and being in joy.
–The Renaissance Women

Time is the space of our lives. It is the circle that encompasses the journey from our birth to our death. Our perception of its passage changes with age and activity. When we were children sitting on the curb in the summer dusk, time dragged by as we waited for the events of our life to unfold. We were small in relationship to time. As the circle of our lives filled with experience time's space shortened. From quiet, endless hours that stretch slowly out before us to blurred weeks that scream by in seconds, we forget that each moment is identical and that time itself has no power to rule us.

Each moment is a gift and each moment is all that we have. Time is our only true possession on this earth, yet we carelessly allow it to fly by, giving it away casually and bestowing it on meaningless objects and events around us.

Taking time means being fully aware. *This* is the only instant in which light shines. Our lives are a full circle to time's closure. Embrace life, appreciate its detail, and celebrate the joy of just being alive. Keep time.

Let us consider things as lent to us.
oh friends: only in passing are we here on earth.
−unknown Aztec Poet

Zen is: Life that knows it is living.
−Frederick Franck

The human race may no longer be able to find meanings, but we have come to understand that we can create them. The notes of the musical scale can be so used and transformed as to become the B-Minor Mass. Paint can become Botticelli's Birth of Venus, with its blowing roses and its goddess of love arising from the sea. Metaphors may become the Vision of God—or intense sexual desire—captured in the image of a white rose unfolding or a red one still in bud.

—Allen Lacy

WHITE ROSE RITUAL

This ritual requires a quantity of white roses and two drops of rose attar or ten drops of rose fragrance. Brew fresh rose-hip tea or make a tisane with one teaspoon of rosewater and one tablespoon of honey stirred into warmed water. Pour this fragrant liquid into your finest cup.

Arrange for an uninterrupted hour and privacy. Serenity is essential to your well-being. Allow the burnished light of late afternoon to enclose your tub or brighten the dusk with a cluster of white candles. Run a tub with pleasantly heated water. As the bath is filling add the fragrance. Drop your robe and sit on the edge of the tub. Pluck the petals from all but one of your bouquet of white roses and launch them upon the water. Lower yourself among the drifting flowers. Slowly sip your warmed tea while the powerful steam works its alchemy.

Become aware of your thoughts and emotions and follow them wherever they wander. When you have finished drinking your tea, pick up the last rose. Clear your mind but of a single image and pull a petal from the flower. Unite petal and image and release both into the water. As the white petal drifts away, let go of the thought embodied in it. With each new petal reach deeper inside yourself and gradually let your thoughts become liquid until no thought is heavier than the rest. Let go of control, accept and trust; reach to clarity and comfort. Everything we relinquish becomes a part of a whole and we float lightly in balance and harmony.

> *Personally creating and thoughtfully selecting the ordinary*
> *things in our daily lives gives them beauty and meaning.*
> *– The Renaissance Women*

CREATING AN ATMOSPHERE OF COMFORT AND WARMTH

Making your bathroom more inviting doesn't have to mean tearing down the walls. There are ways to achieve luxury at little cost. Break the Unwritten Rules of the Bathroom. Rebel against towel racks that pull out of the wall, rug sets designed to disguise the toilet, medicine cabinets that rust, stiff plastic shower curtains, boring soap dish, toothbrush holder, and cup sets, and overwhelming room deodorizers. Treat this room as though you *care* what's in it.

Surround yourself with things that make you feel good. A giant basket of colored towels is a gorgeous sight. Stack or roll them. Choose bath sheets, towels, and robes for texture and size. Quality lasts and you deserve it. Drape them on a freestanding rack, hat tree, or southwestern ladder. Romanticize lighting with candles, colored bulbs, stained-glass kits, and Deco or period lamps. A lighted makeup mirror can change your life and look. Green growing vines, flowering plants, or striking dried arrangements add inexpensive drama. Unusual containers filled with toilet necessities make your bathroom interesting. We use a carved wooden box for cosmetic squares, an onyx dish or crystal salt cellar for pins and rings, a silver cup for cotton swabs, and a Victorian christening mug for toothpaste and brushes.

Display treasures in your bathroom where you will see them every day. Nature's gifts are perfect accessories. Soap is pretty in a seashell or alabaster dish. Sea sponges and loofahs are tubside sculpture. Small changes affect our view of things in more than one way. Water tastes better in a champagne flute, cobalt blue tumbler, or Mickey Mouse glass. Fill your environment with music, books, and magazines. Lean against your bath pillow and admire your artistry.

Recycling is a kindness we give to our burdened planet.
– The Renaissance Women

WRAPPING IT UP

A beautiful package is a gift in itself. Texture, color, and form conspire to arouse our senses even before a gift is opened. Collecting creative gift wrappings and containers is an ongoing scavenger hunt that gives us new perspective. Every day and everywhere we find ordinary and overlooked possibilities.

Antique stores, garage sales, our local grocery, ethnic markets, junk shops, craft suppliers, hardware stores, and building marts all yield uncommon prizes.

Natural elements lend themselves to handmade, personally inspired gifts. The garden, woods, and seashore provide endless resources.

Recycling is a clever way to package gifts economically. Search your office, kitchen, and laundry for reuseables.

Catalogs, magazines, specialty stores, and exclusive shops provide creative suggestions and elegant ideas to adapt for original gift wrappings.

Containers

Baskets; wooden, metal or pottery bowls; shoe boxes, wooden and wine crates; vases; apothecary jars; plastic storage containers; and goblets show off handcrafted gifts. We recycle plastic spray and squeeze bottles; canning jars; mineral water, beer, oil, and vinegar bottles; salsa and spice jars; and jelly glasses.

Coverings

Glue-gun fabric on shoe boxes or baskets. Spray or sponge paint containers. Fabrics, craft papers, and paper bags can be used as they are or decorated with paint, colored pens, or rubber stamps. Dilute white glue with water. Roll a glue-washed bottle or jar top in colored sand, potpourri, seeds, grains, or petals for natural texture. Decoupage boxes or containers with paper cutouts, fabric, lace, or dried botanicals.

Fabric Art

Washcloths, guest towels, handkerchiefs, doilies, napkins, and scarves are ready-made wrappings. Cut squares of lace, tulle, silk, muslin, velvet, felt, and mesh to make bags. Pad jar lids with pillow stuffing and cover with fabric rounds. Tie with ribbon or waxed string.

Attaching

Glue guns are easy to use and provide instant gratification. Everything sticks where it's supposed to. A stapler, ornamental seals and labels, two-sided tape, tacky glue, and a sewing machine are practical tools for gift wrapping.

Wax

Slide string, yarn, or jute through melted wax to make an interesting cord that will hold a shape. Dip bottle tops or corks into wax for a decorative leak-proof seal. Sealing wax can be pressed on a ribbon to secure it around the neck of a bottle or stamped on paper as a handsome seal.

Tying Up

Raffia, waxed string, crochet thread, yarn, ribbon, bead strings, seam bindings and trim, jute, twine, pipe cleaners, lace, French wire ribbon, metallic cord, leather, and shoelaces are great tie-ups.

Tying On

Natural tie-ons include feathers, stones, crystals, cones, pods, seashells, dried flowers, twigs, and berries. Use them directly from nature or spray them in

(continued on page 76)

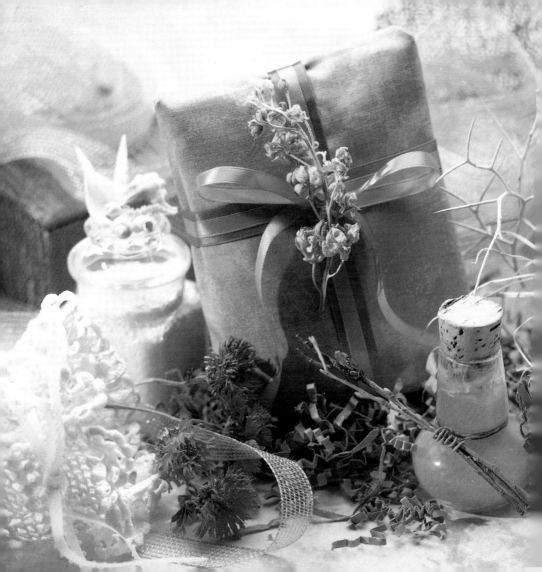

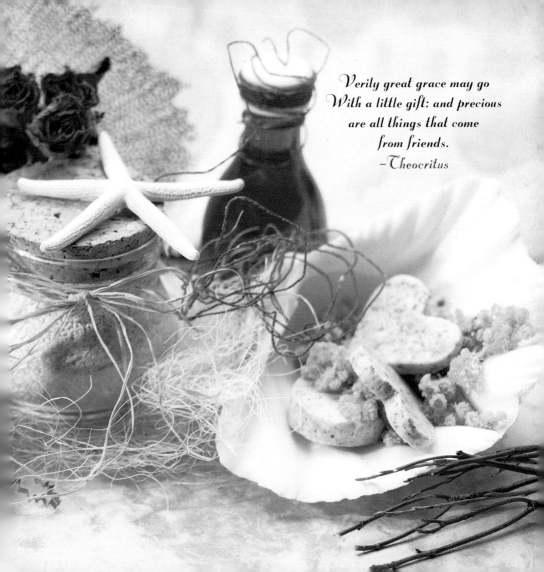

*Verily great grace may go
With a little gift: and precious
are all things that come
from friends.*

—Theocritus

holiday colors. Silk flowers, toys, tokens, bells, beads, and coins can be touched with glitter and paint. Wooden scoops, Oriental soup spoons, and plastic tablespoons are crafty ladles for bath gifts.

Tags and Labels
Make your own personalized computer labels or hand-write on gold and silver foil or ornate paper. Check the catalogs for inexpensive ready-made labels. Cut and recycle greeting cards. Make ceramic tie-ons. Use colored and metallic pens for hand-lettering. Craft stores carry easy-to-use bonding paper to make unique labels with dried botanicals.

Packing
Pack gifts in a bed of shredded paper, wood and straw shavings, colored tissue, potpourri, popcorn, cellophane, dried leaves or grasses.

PACKAGING TECHNIQUES

Fabric Bags
Leak-proof fabric pouches to hold bath products can be made by sewing a plastic Ziploc bag into a square of silk, velvet, brocade, or satin. Calico prints, muslin, or terry cloth have a cozy look, and animal prints delight children.

Cut two pieces of fabric slightly larger than your Ziploc bag. Make one piece four inches longer than the other. With the right sides of the fabric together fold the top edge of the shorter piece over a half inch. Sew three sides to form a pouch. Turn the pouch right-side out and fold the longer edge in two inches. Sew the plastic bag into the opening above its zipper. Press the top flap over like an envelope.

Waxing Bottle Tops and Corks
To make a rich-looking, professional seal, dip a capped or corked bottle in melted wax. Use an old pan you won't need afterward. Beeswax has a mar-

velous aroma. Wax or paraffin may be tinted any color by adding grated crayons to the hot wax.

Fabric Baskets

Commercial fabric stiffener and draping liquid is available at most craft and fabric stores. Soak a long piece of fabric three or four inches wide in stiffener until it is completely saturated. Squeeze out excess liquid. Drape the fabric around the top edge of the basket, tacking with a glue gun to hold. Tie a fabric bow and glue it on the front of the basket. Fabric will hold shape when dry. Fabric containers can be made by placing saturated material over a mold to dry. Try an antique doily, handkerchief, or bandanna.

Metallic Spray Paint

Gold, silver, and copper spray paints turn cones, pods, twigs, seashells, and baskets into gilded art. Their geometry comes alive.

Potpourri Packaging

Wrap bottles or jars in clear cellophane with garden potpourri or dried flowers sprinkled inside. Fill a shallow terra-cotta plant saucer with potpourri and lay your gifts in it. Cover with cellophane and close with a wax seal or colored ribbon.

Ceramic Tie-Ons

Bakeable ceramic clay is available at drugstores and craft shops. Roll and cut it into squares or rounds for labels. Press a design onto the surface with a seashell, cone, or knife. Pierce a hole at the top edge before baking. When cool write a message on the smooth side with a marking pen, and string ribbon or cord through the hole to attach it to a package.

RENAISSANCE...

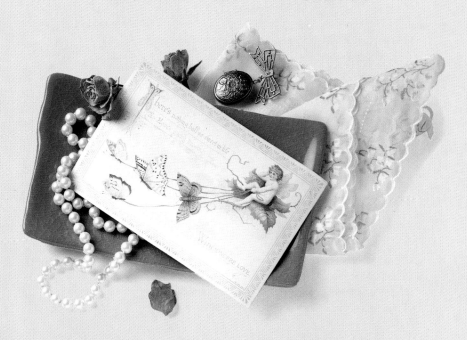

derives from the French word for rebirth and originally referred to the revival of values and the emergence of the artist as a creator. This profound cultural upheaval had its foundation in tradition and learning from the past, enriched by the freedom to revise old rituals.

Our world is experiencing a renaissance to a new age. Women today have the opportunity to weave old lore into new traditions. With our greater resources and unprecedented freedom we are in a unique position to influence the path to the future by supplying value to a chaotic world. We can do this by redefining our relationships with family, friends, society, and the earth.

We are growing to realize that wealth, work, and material possessions do not empower us. We have found that society does not validate the ordinary acts of our daily lives. Many of us undervalue our inner power and stifle our natural talents.

There is a Renaissance woman within us all. It is time to listen to her voice. She has a distinctive style that touches a familiar place in all of us. She takes the time to make each act of giving special. To her love, not perfection, is important. The handmade gifts we receive from her at Christmas, on our birthdays, or sometimes just because we are her friend, are the ones we cherish most.

We all have the capability to unlock our artistic potential and discover the Renaissance woman within. We can create the expensive gifts that we see in stores and catalogs for a fraction of the price and feel appreciated and admired for making them.

Accept disorder with humor. It is a gift to give yourself. Disasters happen! When we were creating formulas for this book, we made some ghastly concoctions and tested them on our families. Support, love, and laughter got us through.

There has never been more reason to learn the art of gifts and giving. We are living on a small planet with limited resources. Using its bounty carefully links us to the earth.

Exercising our creativity opens us to a deepening of emotion and feelings of self-worth. Personal validation is essential no matter who we are or what title we hold. The world cannot and will not validate us; we must do it from within.

PLAN ON IT!

Time passes more quickly than we expect. Full days fly by us without our knowledge or permission. We always plan our Christmas shopping for early summer, but July slides into November and the holidays surprise us every year.

SOURCE GUIDE

Everything you need to make the gifts in this book can be found in local markets, drugstores, or catalogs. We scour the Yellow Pages and find surprises hidden in our own backyards. If you cannot find the supplies you need locally, no problem! Our handy source guide contains reliable mail-order sources around the country for equipment and materials.

GIFT-MAKING SUPPLIES

Alba Naturals, Inc.
P.O. Box 40339
Santa Barbara, CA 93140
800-347-5211
Fax 805-965 0470
unscented bath products

Amrita Aromatherapy, Inc.
P.O. Box 2178
Fairfield, IA 52556
515-472-9136
Fax 515-472-8672
essential oils

Aroma Vera
5901 Rodeo Road
Los Angeles, CA 90016-4312
800-669-9514
Fax 310-280-0395
essential oils, unscented bath products

The Body Shop
45 Horsehill Road
Cedar Knolls, NJ 07927-2014
800-541-2535
fragrance oils, unscented bath products

Body Time
1341 Seventh Street
Berkeley, CA 94710
510-524-0360
Fax 510-527-0979
*fragrance oils, unscented bath
products, bottles*

Caswell-Massey, Co. Ltd.
100 Enterprise Place
Dover, DL 19901
800-326-0500
Fax 800-676-3299
fragrance oils, unscented bath products

Earth Science, Inc.
23705 Via Del Rio
Yorba Linda, CA 92687-2717
800-222-6720
Fax 714-692-8580
unscented bath products

The Essential Oil Company
P.O. Box 206
Lake Oswego, OR 97034
800-729-5912
Fax 503-697-0615
fragrance oils

Essentially Yours of North America
P.O. Box 81866
Bakersfield, CA 93380
805-323-0649
Fax 805-873-7636
essential oils

Essentials & Such
3999 N. Chestnut Diagonal, Suite 368
Fresno, CA 93726-4797
209-298-3313
Fax 209-298-5007
*fragrance oils, unscented bath
products, bottles*

The Fragrant Garden
Portsmouth Road
Erina, NSW 2250 Australia
043 677322
Fax 043-68-1979
fragrance oils, unscented bath products

Herb Products Company
P.O. Box 898
N. Hollywood, CA 91603-0898
213-877-3104
fragrance oils, bulk botanicals

Indiana Botanic Gardens
3401 West Thirty-seventh Avenue
Hobart, IN 46342
219-947-4040
Fax 219-947-4148
fragrance oils, bulk botanicals

Kiehl's, Inc.
109 Third Avenue
New York, NY 10003
800-543-4571
Fax 212-674-3544
fragrance oils

Lavender Lane
6715 Donerail Drive
Sacramento, CA 95842
916-334-4400
Fax 916-339-0842
unscented bath products, bottles

L'Herbier de Provence
462 Seventh Avenue, 17th Floor
New York, NY 10018
212-967-5980
Fax 212-967-5963
fragrance oils, unscented bath products

Leydet Aromatics
P.O. Box 2354
Fair Oaks, CA 95628
916-965-7546
Fax 916-962-3292
essential oils, bottles

Mountain Rose Herbs
P.O. Box 2000
Redway, CA 95560
800-879-3337
Fax 707-923-7867
*unscented bath products, bottles,
bulk botanicals*

Original Swiss Aromatics
P.O. Box 6842
San Rafael, CA 94903
415-459-3998
essential oils

Santa Fe Fragrance Consultants
P.O. Box 282
Santa Fe, NM 87504
Phone and Fax 505-473-1717
essential oils

The Ultimate Herb
& Spice Shoppe
111 Azalea, Box 395
Duenweg, MO 64841
417-782-0457
fragrance oils, bulk botanicals

Uncommon Scents
P.O. Box 1941
Eugene, OR 97440-1941
800-426-4336
Fax 503-343-8196
*fragrance oils, unscented bath
products, bottles*

BATH AND BEAUTY GIFTS

Abracadabra, Inc.
P.O. Box 1040
Guerneville, CA 95446
800-745-0761
Fax 707-869-9367

Comptoir Sud Pacifique
331 Poinciana Plaza
Palm Beach, FL 33480
407-820-9020
Fax 407-820-9222

Essentiel Elements
2415 Third Street, Suite 235
San Francisco, CA 94107
415-621-9881
Fax 415-621-6977

Essence AromaTherapy
P.O. Box 2119
Durango, CO 81301
800-283-0244
Fax 303-247-0118

Floris
703 Madison Avenue
New York, NY 10021
800-535-6747
Fax 212-888-2001

Moon River Naturals
886 W. Sixth Street, Suite B
Eugene, OR 97402
503-687-8339

Rémy Laure
11281 Interchange Circle South
Miramar, FL 33025
800-255-7369
Fax 305-438-6841

Zia Cosmetics
410 Townsend Street, 2nd Floor
San Francisco, CA 94107
800-334-7546
Fax 415-543-7694

LUXURY BATH ACCESSORIES

Chambers
P.O. Box 7841
San Francisco, CA 94120-7841
800-334-9790
Fax 415-421-5153

Crabtree & Evelyn
P.O. Box 158
Woodstock, CT 06281-0158
800-272-2873
Fax 203-928-0828

Cuddledown of Maine
312 Canco Road
P.O. Box 1910
Portland, ME 04104-1910
800-323-6793
Fax 207-761-1948

Horchow
P.O. Box 620048
Dallas, TX 75262-0048
800-456-7000
Fax 214-401-6414

QUOTE PERMISSION AND ACKNOWLEDGMENTS

Thinking Like a Mountain, John Seed and Joanna Macy, © 1988.
New Society Publishers.

Everyday Wisdom, Dr. Wayne W. Dyer, © 1993. Hay House, Inc., Carson, CA.
Used by permission.

To Dance with God, Gertrud Mueller Nelson, © 1986. Paulist Press.

A Stone, A Leaf, A Door, Thomas Wolfe, © 1973. Paul Gitlin, administrator,
Estate of Thomas Wolfe.

The Grandmother of Time, Zsuzsanna Emese Budapest, © 1989.
HarperCollins.

The Zen of Seeing, Frederick Franck, © 1973. Random House.

The Feminine Face of God, Sherry Ruth Anderson and Patricia Hopkins,
© 1991. Bantam. By permission of authors.

Truth or Dare, Starhawk, © 1987 by Miriam Simos. HarperCollins.

Blood Memory, Martha Graham, © 1991. Doubleday.

The Mythic Image, Joseph Campbell, © 1974. Princeton University Press.

The Glory of Roses, © 1990 Allen Lacy and Christopher Baker. Reprinted
by permission of Stewart, Tabori & Chang, Publishers.

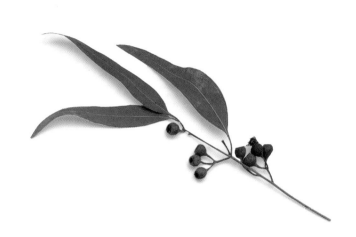